CORA WISHER

ALTERNATIVE MEDICINE

**The Ultimate Guide to the Healing Benefits of
Alternative Medicine, Discover All the Information
About Non-Traditional Healing**

Descrierea CIP a Bibliotecii Naționale a României
CORA WISHER
   ALTERNATIVE MEDICINE. The Ultimate Guide to the Healing Benefits of Alternative Medicine, Discover All the Information About Non-Traditional Healing / Cora Wisher – Bucharest: Editura My Ebook, 2020
   ISBN

CORA WISHER

ALTERNATIVE MEDICINE
The Ultimate Guide to the Healing Benefits of Alternative Medicine, Discover All the Information About Non-Traditional Healing

My Ebook Publishing House
Bucharest, 2020

TABLE OF CONTENTS

INTRODUCTION

Traditionally, the first response for Americans to any type of medical issue is conventional medicine. There is, however, another option. Alternative medicine is sometimes considered the oldest medicine in the world.

Alternative medicine envelops the concept of seeking out non-traditional ways to deal with day-to-day health issues. This type of medicine looks beyond taking medication.

People look to use alternative medicine for two main reasons. The first is because of the idea that taking medications can potentially lead to unhealthy results such as dependencies and side effects. The second is because of the natural curiosity of man to find better methods to heal.

Alternative medicine encompasses many different therapies, such as hypnosis, color therapy, yoga, meditation, herbal remedies, vitamin therapy, and many more.

The main focus of alternative medicine is that life is a combination of parts that includes more than the treatment of disease. There is a definite focus on living life well, happily, and with purpose. It is believed that this is an essential part of healthy living.

This guide will explore the many different components of alternative medicine, and how it can help you. Consider using the ideas captured here next time you feel ill to begin feeling better naturally.

CHAPTER 1

ALTERNATIVE MEDICINE & ITS HISTORY

Treatments Beyond Conventional

When most people get sick, they look to conventional methods of medical treatment for relief and healing. There are alternative methods to treatment that are becoming increasingly popular.

What treatments are considered "conventional?" Prescription medication, traditional surgery, and computerized scientific testing are three examples of conventional medicine. Most physicians support conventional medicine in their practices, so when seeing a doctor, it is highly likely you will be advised to follow conventional medical advise.

The decision to use conventional medicine should be made by the patient and doctor on a case by case basis. An alteration to the type of treatment is sometimes all that is needed to feel better.

Alternative treatments include:

Herbal remedies

Massage

Meditation

Acupuncture

Many more!

Patients will often find themselves turning to alternative methods of treatment when conventional methods are ineffective or a medical problem has been deemed untreatable. Alternative treatments are designed to not only aid in pain relief, but also reduce stress and tension that can worsen chronic pain.

Alternative methods of treatment focus on the whole person; body and soul. Convention methods strictly focus on the physical problems alone. For alternative methods to be effective, the patient must be motivated and believe in the alternative treatment's ability to work.

Of course, any serious, life-threatening health problem should blend conventional and alternative methods for a comprehensive approach. Be sure to consult with your doctor to avoid complications. If planned well, you can take advantage of best of both types of medicine for a life that is comfortable and enjoyable.

Alternative Medicine History & Theory

Thousands of years ago, all medicine was "alternative medicine." Before modern science, healers would consider the full picture - emotional, physical, and spiritual – before healing a sick person.

This is one of the main differences between modern conventional medicine and alternative medicine. Alternative medicine does not look for the instant cure for the physical problem, rather is looks more at a long-term solution that includes the whole self.

Just a few centuries ago in Europe there were two types of healers; folk healers that used old tried-and-true methods, and professional physicians. The lower classes did not have the money to pay for the professional physicians, but they used the folk healers and it worked.

In North America, philosophy and religion were often used to help folk healers provide holistic treatments.

The conventional medicine that we have today has evolved from the days of folk healers and alternative medicine. Many conventional physician support different types of holistic treatments in the overall wellness plan for their patients. The reason that alternative medicine has stood the test of time is because it works!

Ancient Chinese Medicine

Traditional Chinese medicine (TCM) includes acupuncture, Qigong, herbal treatments, deep massage, and more. More than 25% of the world's population practices TCM.

Several reputable groups, such as the World Health Organization and the National Institute of Health, find traditional Chinese medicine to be a viable alternative to contemporary medicine.

Many parts of TCM began well over 3,000 years ago in China. The focus of TCM is Qi (pronounced "Chee"), which is the body's energy that connects it to the world around us. It is believed that all disorders and bodily problems are caused by the misalignment of Qi. Acupuncture is one of the most widely recognized methods of bringing the Qi into alignment.

Herbal remedies are popular in traditional Chinese medicine. They are used to relax and calm the patient's emotions to avoid depression, and provide a more positive outlook on the illness. This helps tremendously in the healing process. Ginseng and herbal green tea are the most popular herbal remedies in China.

Exercise, mainly Qigong (pronounce "Chee Kung"), is also an important part of traditional Chinese medicine. Qigong involves posture, meditation, and slow, calculated body movements.

Tibetan Medicine

Tibetan Medicine is almost solely based on herbal remedies, and has been around for over 2,500 years. It is called "gSoba Rig-pa". Tibetans mostly live in India because they have been in exile since the late 1950's. They practice Tibetan Buddhism.

There is a Tibetan Medical Institute in Northern India, where doctors studying Tibetan medicine attend for 7 years before earning a degree.

The underlying belief in Tibetan medicine is that all illnesses are caused by poisonous thinking which include dread, denial, and want. This concept ties to the principles of Buddhist philosophy.

The three poisonous thoughts are believed to be caused by poor diet, inappropriate behavior, and the imbalance of time and season. This concept is more complicated than this, but this simplification will give a general sense of it.

Cures are linked to all systems of the body working together. The elimination of sweat, feces and urine contributes to this harmony.

Similar to the Chinese "Qi", the Tibetans have the Rlung, which is the overall life force that connects us to the universe. Rlung has five types:

1. Centered in the brain. Life grasping – controls breathing, intellect, sneezing and swallowing.

2. Centered in the chest. Upward moving – controls verbal ability and stamina.

3. Centered in the heart. All pervading – controls all movement like that of the orifices of the body and walking.

4. Centered in the stomach. Fire accompanying – controls digestion and metabolism.

5. Centered in the rectum. Downward cleansing – controls everything that is expelled from the body, such as babies, menstrual blood or semen.

Tibetan medicine usually handles sickness diagnosis by analysis of the tongue and urine. The spiritual element is also at play in Tibetan medicine, with much attention spent focusing on the type and temperament of spirits in the body.

American Indian Medicine (aka Native American Medicine)

North American Indian tribes have been practicing medicine for what some claim to be over 40,000 years. The medical information and techniques are handed down from generation to generation; ensure the longevity of the practice.

Some remedies are tribe-specific, although all tribal medicine is called Native American Medicine, collectively. Native Americans believe that man is one with nature and that the elements provide strength and can cure disease.

It is fascinating to note that at the same time that Native American medicine was being practiced in North America, Traditional Chinese Medicine was being practiced a half a world away. Ayurveda (medicine practiced in India), was also practiced at this time, and will be covered next.

All of these traditional medical practices are based on the same fundamental belief that a person's lifestyle and environment should be taken into consideration before choosing a treatment path. There are subtle differences between the practices that are specific to the region.

Native American medicine recognizes a purification procedure involving herbal smoke before and after treatment. Treatments include the use of sage and cedar smoke to repel negative energy. Negative energy is considered the pain released by someone who is ill, or the pain that the healer takes on themselves from their patients. Therapeutic touch is used. Singing, chanting, drums and rattles accompany the healing during the session.

Ayurvedic Medicine

Ayurvedic Medicine is practiced in India, and focuses on natural healing. Practitioners believe that it is important for the body to be balanced, and all medicines are based on vegetables and minerals, with the active ingredients from plant alkaloids.

In Ayurvedic Medicine there is the belief that there are three elements in the body, called Kapha, Pitta, and Vata, that cause disease.

1. Kapha: This energy is caused by the lack of stabilizing the balance in the body. These are commonly called viruses by Westerners.

2. Pitta: This energy supports vision, temperature, hunger, thirst, intelligence, and happiness. When out of alignment, the outcomes include weight fluctuation, dehydration, depression, digestive issues, and apathy.

3. Vata: This energy keeps the overall balance between the earth, sky and world around us in check with ourselves. If it falls out of balance, sickness is invited in.

Disease is called Vyaadhi, and it is treated by focusing on the imbalance of elements.

CHAPTER 2

ALTERNATIVE TREATMENT OPTIONS

Homeopathy Treatments

Homeopathy is defined as an organic system of medicine that is based on three main ideas:

1. Like cures like
2. Minimal dosing
3. One time remedies

Alternative medicine traditionally has the least amount of "active" ingredient possible, with the concept of using one single remedy irregardless of how many symptoms are presenting. Homeopathy focuses on the least amount of treatments for better health.

There are several reasons why homeopathy is the second most popular form of medicine (after conventional medicine). The most popular reasons are:

It is extremely natural and safe

The results are permanent

It is effective

You can take most homeopathic medicines along with conventional medicine without side effects

It is non-addictive

Homeopathy is a precise science, which is why it sometimes takes longer to find exactly the right medicine for your illness. Alternative medicine spends time asking questions about symptoms and the root cause of the illness in an effort to make a clear diagnosis for the problem, and treat it effectively.

Herbal Remedies

Nature provides many cures and treatments for ailments of all kinds. Each region has its own native plants that are used in alternative medicine.

When buying herbs for medicinal purposes, it is suggested that you use herbs from an herbal shop. Herb strength varies depending on the way in which they are grown, so until you are familiar with growing techniques for medicinal herbs, purchasing from a professional is recommended.

The following list provides herbal cures to common ailments:

Acne and skin blemishes.

Wash your face and rub a clove of garlic that has been cut in half. Or, mix lavender with witch hazel at a 1:10 ratio. Tea tree oil can be substituted in place of the lavender.

Anxiety and stress.

Lavender pure essential oil soaked onto a cotton cloth, heated, and folded into a compress. Apply to head or neck.

Bruises and contusions.

Boil hyssop flowers and leaves into a tincture. Filter liquid, and soak a cotton compress. Apply to bruised area by applying pressure. The hyssop, heat and pressure combination will reduce the bruise.

Burns.

Minor burns can be treated with comfrey or aloe juice. Simply rub aloe juice into burned area. Comfrey can be crushed into a fine powder, mixed with equal parts of melted beeswax, and added to vegetable oil. Simmer over low heat for 20 minutes, and then strain mixture.

Warts.

Either use a cut piece of garlic, placed directly on the wart or, for a less odorous cure, try dandelion juice applied repeatedly throughout the day.

Herbal Teas

An age old remedy, herbal teas are used to soothe and relive pain and stress. Many teas are actually a *tincture* rather than a tea. A tincture is a thicker tea that is herb-dense and is infused instead of steeped.

The following list is a list of conditions and herbal tea remedies:

Anemia.

Drink a tincture made from boiled stinging nettle leaves.

Arthritis.

Drink a tincture of devil's claw, juniper, birch, or celery seed (not the type on your spice rack).

Chemotherapy side effects.

Drink a tincture of Siberian ginseng root. It soothes the insides and relieves fatigue.

Colic in babies.

Add less than 10 drops of dill and fennel tincture to their bottle.

Constipation.

Drink a liter of rhubarb root per day.

Cough.

Drink a tea made from garlic bulbs and ribwort leaves.

Depression.

Drink a tincture daily made from the ground up oat plant and St. John's wart flowers.

Fever.

Drink a hot tea made of lemon balm, yarrow, and ginger.

Gas.

Drink a tea made of caraway, fennel, ginger, and peppermint.

Flu symptoms.

Drink a tincture made of Echinacea, yarrow, and catnip.

Vitamins & Minerals

Taking a vitamin supplement is not a substitution for eating healthfully. However, it does serve as insurance to be certain that you are getting all of the vitamins and minerals that your body needs.

Vitamins are essential to the optimized functioning of your body. Without sufficient vitamins, for example, your blood will not clot. You need vitamins to fight colds, and boost your immune system.

It is best to take a homeopathic test to determine the vitamins that you need. This will avoid a dangerous overdose. Then you can take the vitamins you need individually, as needed, and avoid a multi-vitamin, which is chockfull of fillers.

This method will save you money, too.

Bee Therapy (aka Apitherapy)

The practice of Apitherapy is the use of bee stings, bee pollen, propolis, royal jelly, and honey to treat a variety of aliments. While there has not been extensive testing in the scientific world to validate the claims of apitherapists, history proves that the treatments provide relief.

There are five honeybee products that are used in apitherapy:

1. **Venom**: A practitioner will aid the patient in injecting or being stung by bees in the affected area. The venom is used to provide relief for conditions such as tendonitis, Multiple Sclerosis, and degenerative bone disease. It works because the venom is a natural anti-inflammatory which is more potent then others available to conventional medicine such as hydrocortisone. You must get tested to be certain that you are not allergic to beestings prior to exposing yourself to bee venom.

2. **Pollen**: A natural energy supplement that is also used as a seasonal allergy aid. It is also believed to slow down the development of wrinkles.

3. **Raw Honey**: A source of quick energy, raw honey is used for many cures. It can even be used as a salve on top of an open wound to avoid the spread of bacteria.

4. **Royal Jelly**: Is the milky white substance that the worker bees produce to feed the queen. While unsubstantiated, this substance is used as a beauty aid and is believed to help lower cholesterol.

5. **Propolis**: Is the glue used to keep the hives together and make repairs. Propolis is made from the sap of poplar and

24

conifer trees. It is used to make lip balm and salves, and is considered to be an antioxidant.

Iridology

Iridology is name for the practice of determining a person's toxicity based on the color of their iris. This concept goes back to Sweden and Hungary where physicians used it to gauge disease in their patients.

For centuries, famous physicians and scientists, all the way back to the Greek physician Hippocrates, have found the people with injuries get black marks across the iris of their eye. These marks later disappear as the person's ailments heal.

In today's world, iridology is used as a preventative measure to gauge if there is a change in a person's health. It is unfortunate that iridology cannot be used to identify a specific disease.

The way in which iridology is practiced today is that the colored part of the eye (the iris) is carefully photographed using a strong camera lens. It is painless, and it takes about an hour to complete. The photos are then enlarged, and a trained professional iridologist studies it for signs of possible illness.

Even conventional doctors use the eyes as an early warning sign of bad things going on inside of the body. This study is just the more focused analysis of the iris when looking for signs of degenerative health issues.

Meditation in Healing

Meditation is a skill that is learned. Once you know how to do it properly, it can be used to greatly improve your quality of life and health.

The benefits of meditation are an increased level of energy, a more positive attitude, a better immune health, better sleep quality, and the slowing of the aging process.

To take advantage of the maximum benefit, meditate for at least 20 minutes per day prior to bedtime.

Follow these steps for meditating. First, sit down and get comfortable in a quiet room. Keep your back and neck straight, and clear your mind so that you are focusing on the present moment.

Then become aware of your breathing. Breathe in and out of your mouth, and pay attention to your stomach rising and falling.

If thoughts come into your head, acknowledge them and let the pass through your mind. Remain conscious of your breathing and relax. If your thoughts carry you away, don't get frustrated. Simply return back to focusing on your breathing.

When your time meditating is finished, become aware of your surroundings and stand up slowly.

Meditation is a wonderful way to instantly relax yourself and reenter your being. It is the perfect supplement to any treatment, both alternative and contemporary.

This deep relaxation technique will help remove stress and anxiety from life. Reduced stress can only help healing.

Tai Chi & Yoga

Tai Chi is a very gentle form of exercise that anyone can do. Since most people spend most of their time sitting, it is imperative that regular exercise become a part of their daily routine. Tai Chi can become that daily movement.

Exercise helps by improving circulatory function, reducing headache tension, lowering blood pressure, and eliminating chronic back and neck pain.

Tai Chi is a series of movements and stretches that anyone can do from any position, even sitting. The exercise will improve posture, stamina, and flexibility.

Movements in Tai Chi are slow and deliberate, and easy to learn. Attending a class is the best way to learn Tai Chi. Do not worry about not being in shape; Tai Chi is known to be an exercise that is done by all types of people, of all ages.

Yoga

Yoga is a great exercise activity for all types of people. It is not difficult, but you do have to want to learn about it. The main goal of yoga is to create a balanced relationship between you physical and mental health.

Yoga is a way of life that is carried throughout the day, not just while in yoga class. Yoga creates an awareness of yourself and your day to day life. This is a drastic change to many people who often live on autopilot.

You can decide how you want to use yoga, for its basic purpose of bringing together mind and body, or as more of a strenuous activity for exercise purposes.

In yoga, it is best to start out at the lowest level possible and work your way up as you develop strength and understanding. Just like most other things, it is important to know the foundational concepts before branching out into more difficult territory,

You can take instructor-led classes, or learn at home through the wide variety of DVDs.

Birkram Yoga

Birkram yoga is also known as "hot yoga", mainly because it is practiced in a space that has been heated to over 115 degrees. Hot yoga mainly focuses on stretches and balance. It also is filled with moves that create pressure in the body that blocks circulation. By going through the movements, the constant build up of pressure created by stretching are then released, providing a rush of blood through the veins. This is believed to clean them out.

There are 26 poses in hot yoga. The purpose for the hot environment in Birkram yoga is the warmth warms the body's muscles and tendons which aids in flexibility.

There are a few tips for people considering this type of yoga. First, because it is practiced in a hot room, you will sweat a lot. It is best to wear appropriate light clothing. It is also a good idea to drink plenty of water prior to your session.

Hatha Yoga

The main focus of Hatha yoga is breathing, meditation, and posture. The practice of this form of yoga is perfect for people that are new to it. Hatha yoga has more of a strong emphasis on the mental component of meditation, mixed in with yoga.

Karma Yoga

The Karma form of yoga pulls together the spiritual and physical worlds. The fundamentals of Karma yoga are based in the Hindu philosophy and religion. It combines two competing philosophies in the world; from the West – that life should be pleasure based, and from the East – that life should be lived for knowledge. Both theories are blended in karma.

Your karma growth is dependant on how you live your life. Bad karma comes from living your life for the purpose of money, wealth, and material possessions. Good karma comes from living your life for happiness and love.

Karma yoga helps you focus on your life as you learn about you life goals, and helps guide you in the right direction.

Neuro Linguistic Programming (NLP)

Neuro Linguistic Programming can be considered the power of positive thought and prayer. It is well documented throughout science and medicine that having a positive attitude, outlook, and having a positive support system surround you is one of the most effective alternative medicines available.

NLP is a method of programming your thoughts in order to be positive. This technique focuses on your sub-conscious and your dreams. It is imperative to truly believe that you can heal yourself for NLP to work.

How do you practice NLP? First, take a strategy that you know creates success in other areas of your life, and apply it to your healing process. You absolutely must have faith in your body's healing ability for this to work.

Muscular and Skeletal Alternative Medicine

There are numerous other alternative treatments for the skeletal and muscular systems of the body. They include:

1. Kinesiology

Professionals test the various muscles throughout the body to determine areas that are not balanced properly, and then restore balance by using a variety of techniques.

2. Rolfing

Rolfing is the use of pressure to massage the connective tissue within the body. This allows for the body to be more flexible and be aligned properly. Rolfing will provide more energy and less anxiety.

3. Massage Therapy

Massage therapy is used to break up the knotted muscles, and to retrain the muscles. It works the ligaments, tendons, and soft tissue muscles. Massage therapy increases circulation and improves breathing.

4. Color therapy

Color therapy uses color and light to treat ailments. Often considered a complementary treatment, color therapy is used in addition to other treatment.

There are seven colors that correspond to the wavelength centers of the body. Each color is matched with a region of the body.

5. Magnetic energy

The use of magnetic energy fields to, as magnetic therapists believe, to manipulate cells with magnetic energy. They also believe they can recharge cells. Magnetic energy can also increase blood flow that will then reduce scars on organs, provide migraine relief, and other reoccurring pain.

6. Craniosacral therapy (CST)

The craniosacral system is the membranes and fluid that envelopes the brain and spinal cord. By applying gentle pressure to the head, the rhythm of the cranioscaral system can be evaluated and in some ways manipulated. This improves the flow and function of the central nervous system. This treatment is used in alternative medicine as a preventative measure. Professional craniosacral therapy practitioners believe they can locate and release energy cysts by unblocking them and realigning the neck.

Acupuncture

In acupuncture, thin needles are inserted into the skin to draw nerve stimulation at pinpointed locations around the body. Acupuncture is a Chinese medical procedure that involves Dao – the advocate for living in balance and moderation, with ying and yang – two life elements that are apposing forces that when balanced brings good health and happiness. Acupuncture brings relief of pain, aids respiratory illnesses, and relieves headaches and ulcers, among other physical issues. It also balances the qi life force.

Reiki

Reiki is the practice of transferring healing energy from the healer's hands to the ill person. This can be done hands-on and from a distance. The healer is believed to be full of universal energy. It is thought that the practitioner can use Reiki energy to alter the frequency of the aura. Healing is achieved first physically, then emotionally, and finally spiritually.

Crystals: A Tool for Healing

Crystals have long been associated with alternative healing. A crystal is created when crystalline is formed by minerals being arranged in a precise pattern.

Quartz is the most popular crystal. The belief behind the use of crystals is that blocked energy will be released when the crystal is placed at specific points around the body.

CHAPTER 3

OVERALL TREATMENT PLANS &
ADDITIONAL TIPS

Five Ways to Bring the Mind, Body & Spirit Together

Mind and body are easily defined, but what is the "spirit" of you? The spirit, or soul, can be considered the part of you that is spiritually passionate. What makes you passionate? Here are a few ideas that can help you decide:

1. Look forward to something that you can anticipate.

2. Create a happy place where you can go when you meditate.

3. Reminisce about your successes.

4. Find something that relieves your stress and do it.

5. Explore your future goals – not money related.

Kama-Sutra

The Kama-Sutra is ancient text about sexual health that was written sometime between the 1st and 6th century in India. There are 35 chapters that cover everything from how to find a wife, to how to perform in bed, to how to make yourself attractive to others.

Sections of the book cover the relationship between diet and sexual wellbeing. Wholesome, nutritious foods are specifically referenced. Histamines are recommended, through food, for increased sexual pleasure.

Breathing techniques are stressed. This helps ease stress and improves overall sexual health.

Feng Shui

Feng Shui is the concept of bring nature and natural patterns and surroundings into our homes and everyday lives. This will bring harmony and peaceful alignment with the world.

Feng Shui brings together all of the elements. Fire, earth, air, and water, and the additional "metal", are represented inside the home by the selection of lighting, scents, sounds, and the placement of furniture and fixtures.

The underlying concept is that the qi, or life force, must be able to move freely in a room. Therefore, the location of furniture, for example, is important.

Chiropractics

Chiropractics is an alternative medicinal practice that is now considered conventional. The main theory behind chiropractics is that the vertebrate of the spine is not in alignment. It is believed that this misalignment causes many diseases and disorders throughout the body.

Chiropractors use pressure to realign and adjust the spine. Most chiropractors also look at the whole picture – stress, lifestyle choices, and overall health – when recommending treatment.

Chiropractors have been known to heal a wide range of medical problems through their work on patient's backs. Asthma, migraines, arthritis and more issues can all be positively impacted.

This treatment is safe and usually inexpensive. It is non-evasive. Going to a chiropractor will certainly require regular visits because your issues will not be fully treated in just one session.

Biofeedback

Biofeedback is a tool used to gauge internal function, then determine treatment, and then gauge if treatment is working properly. Similar to a thermometer or scale to measure the body weight or if there is a fever, biofeedback is garnered through tools.

The body function that it is measuring is activity that one cannot voluntarily control, such as blood pressure and brain wavelengths.

The main recommendation in alternative health for biofeedback is usually relaxation. This reduces the heart rate, calms the brain, and greatly impacts the affected parts of the body.

Using Alternative Medicine in Children

Sometimes conventional treatments are not an option for children. One example of when alternative medicines are a viable option for children is when they refuse to take their over-the-counter medication. They might be more willing to take an herbal remedy because it is something different.

Consider discussing with your conventional doctor these supplementary treatments for children:

Acupuncture

The needles release endorphins to the brain which can help kids with asthma, and reduce other pains.

Hypnosis

This technique might give a child more discipline regarding the regular administration of their conventional medication.

Relaxation techniques and massage

This can help kids with asthma deal with constricting airways. Massage can help relax the stress surround asthma as well. Breathing techniques can help kids feel in control of their breathing. Kids with more serious diseases such as diabetes and cancer can use the relaxing benefits of massage to relieve stress and help maintain a positive outlook.

Always do plenty of research and consult with your child's doctor before beginning any alternative medical techniques.

Gender-Specific Alternative Medicine

Men and women each have their own medical needs specific to their gender. It is wise to consider what areas of alternative medicine are best geared for your gender.

For women, issues related to menstruation – such as regular menstruation and PMS are always hot topics. For these issues, women have the following homeopathic options:

Acupuncture

Chinese medicinal herbs & herbal teas

Osteopathy

Crystal therapy

Yoga

Hypnosis

For men, issues around prostate health and overall wellbeing can involve an alternative approach. Men have these choices:

Yoga

Acupuncture

Herbal treatments

Men and women both need to care for their health. A proactive, homeopathic approach will ensure a happy, healthy life.

Homeopathic Weight Loss

There are alternative techniques that can be used in the fight to lose unwanted pounds. Of course, just like in conventional medicine, there is no magic pill.

However, the standard "eat well, be more active" technique of losing weight can be enhanced with alternative medicine.

First, you can consider yoga. This exercise is slow and calculated, but the results can be dramatic. When practices wholeheartedly and regularly, you can gain muscle and lose fat.

Acupuncture can reduce food cravings that are sabotaging your weight loss efforts. Teas can help curb cravings as well as detoxify the body.

Follow these tips to lose weight with alternative medicine:

1. Use a juicer to drink your fruits and vegetables.

2. Add Omega-3 to your beverages.

3. Visit a homeopathic doctor for a nutritional evaluation.

4. Contact an herbalist for recommendations on alternative teas.

5. Consider taking bovine or shark cartilage.

6. Hypnosis can be used for behavioral modification.

Alternative Medicine and Cancer

People with cancer often look for viable options that they can use to fight this disease. Unfortunately, there is no cure for cancer. Conventional treatments are the most aggressive, and while alternative and conventional medicine should work together to provide a comprehensive medical experience, at this time they do not.

You can use alternative medicine to supplement your conventional cancer treatments. Here are some of the best complementary alternative treatments:

1. Acupuncture: Helps with nausea, tiredness, pain, headaches.

2. Herbal remedies: Ginger, for one, is helpful in dealing with nausea and vomiting caused by chemotherapy.

3. Hyperbaric oxygen therapy is currently being studies as a complementary treatment for radiation therapy.

4. Massage helps relieve fatigue.

One of the biggest benefits of complimentary treatments is that the sick person can take control over their situation and treatment, even if just in a small way. This helps the patient's chances for survival and improves the quality of life.

As with any medical treatment, consult with your doctor before self-treating. Dangerous and counterproductive side effects can result if treatment is not cohesively planned.

What Happens in an Alternative Treatment Session?

First and foremost, it is essential to pick the right practitioner for you. When selecting your perfect practitioner, be sure to review their credentials because there are many fraudulent practitioners in the alternative medical world.

Follow these tips to find the perfect practitioner:

1. Search the phone book and online for local professionals. Select alocal group of practitioners.

2. Research this group of practitioners to find out their experience, education, style, and anything else you can about them.

3. Find out what organizations they are affiliated with. The more trade groups, the better.

4. Contact them to ask what specific experience they have with your type of situation.

5. Ask what the treatment process is for your given situation.

The focus of an alternative medicine session is different then what occurs in a conventitional medical session. Here, the practitioner will want to learn about you as a whole person, not just the specific area of injury or concern.

How to Become an Alternative Medical Practitioner

Are you thinking about becoming an alternative medical practitioner? The profession is rewarding and interesting, and provides you with the opportunity to help people. By providing an alternative medicine service, you will be making a difference in the world.

First, you will need to determine which type of alternative medicine you want to practice. Alternative medicine is broken down into seven categories:

1. Dioelectricmagnetic applications
2. Diet
3. Nutrition

4. Lifestyle changes

5. Herbal medicine

6. Manual healing

7. Biological treatments

To become a professional alternative medicine practitioner, you will need to successfully complete an accredited program at a registered school. There are many schools that specialize in one area or another of alternative medicine.

Schooling is intensive, and a good program will include years of study and practice, as well as an internship experience.

Once you have completed school and practicum work you will be able to practice your field of study on your own.

Paying for Alternative Medicine

Prices for alternative treatments vary. Most treatments are not covered by insurance, so it is important to discuss actual costs prior to rendering services from a practitioner.

The first step in finding out how to pay for treatment is to call your insurance company to see if they will cover your treatment session. If they do cover, find out the specifics. How many sessions? Is there a specific type of treatment that is only covered?

When you meet your practitioner, one of the first questions to ask is if they accept your type of insurance. If you are not using insurance, you will need to work out alternative payment.

CONCLUSION

In North America, alternative medicine has experienced an increase in popularity in recent years. Of course, there is controversy surrounding the two big types of medicine; conventional and traditional.

With all of the wonderful benefits of alternative medicine, there are some risks associated with it. The follow risks should be considered before using alternative medicine:

1. Unsafe, ineffective, untested substances

2. Listening to exaggerated claims of safety by some unscrupulous businesses

3. Forgoing conventional treatments for serious illnesses to use an alternative treatment.

4. Not disclosing the simultaneous use of both conventional and alternative treatments, possibly creating a negative health situation

It is important to recognize possible risks in alternative medicine. As with anything, if a therapy, product or substance sound like it is too good to be true – then it probably is!

Always research the therapy or substance, as well as any practitioners that you are thinking about using. Check credentials and references, if possible. Because much of the alternative medicine world is unregulated, there are frauds out there that you will need to be weary of.

If you are careful about what you put in your body, and the types of external therapy you solicit, you can make educated choices that will benefit your health greatly.

The best approach is a strategically planned approach that you create and discuss with your doctor. If you are not comfortable talking with your conventional medical doctor about supplementing with alternative medicine treatments, then find one that is open mined about this type of treatment. You will be happy you did.

Only once you have research all the different alternative treatments from around the world will you have a full understanding about what options are actually out there. The internet is an excellent place to begin your research journey.

Printed by Libri Plureos GmbH in Hamburg,
Germany